# Your Guru Guide to Breaking into the Hair Industry

By Eryka Monson

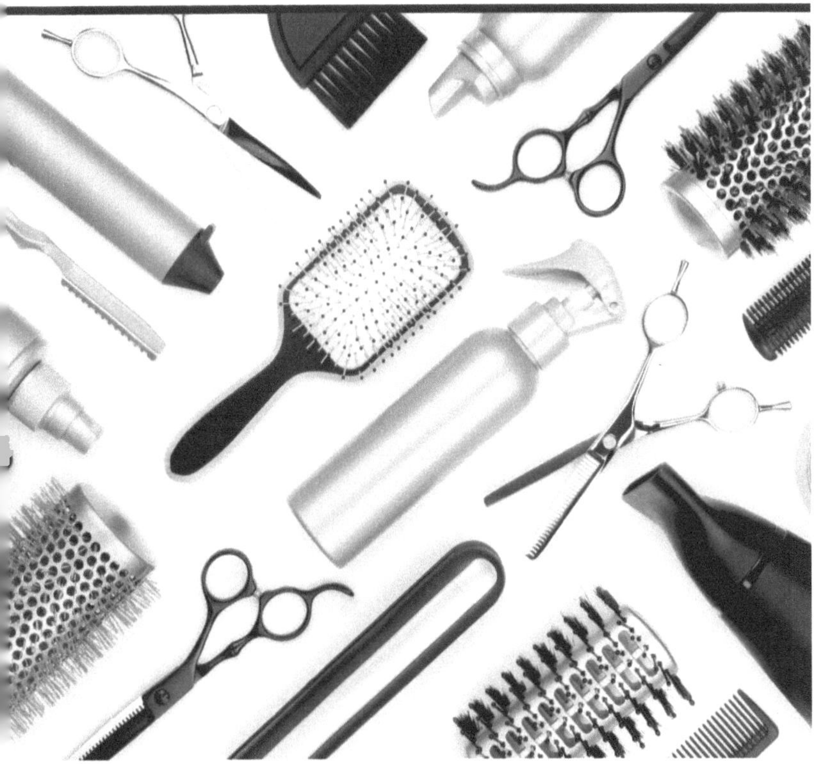

# Table of Contents

INTRODUCTION

# Hi, I'm Eryka.

I'm so excited to help guide and direct new, up and coming, and even seasoned stylists on the lifelong journey with the hair industry.

Some background about who I am and why I am wirting this guide: in short, I learned some tips and tricks that others didn't seem to be doing, and wanted to pass that forward, because I am at a time in my life that I can no longer devote the same time or energy, either physically or emotionally into the industry that has treated me so well.

I love being able to transform and impact women and men's lives when they come and sit in my chair. I am as much a therapist as I am a stylist. I am as much a friend and confidant as I am a necessary part of their personal beauty maintenance.

As a seasoned stylist with 20+ years of experience, I've seen firsthand the transformative power of hair styling not just on my clients' appearances, but also on their confidence and self-esteem. The journey from aspiring stylist to successful business owner is a challenging yet incredibly rewarding one. I'm excited to share my insights, experiences and some of my top secrets in earning and maintaining a 6-figure income from behind the chair with you in this ebook.

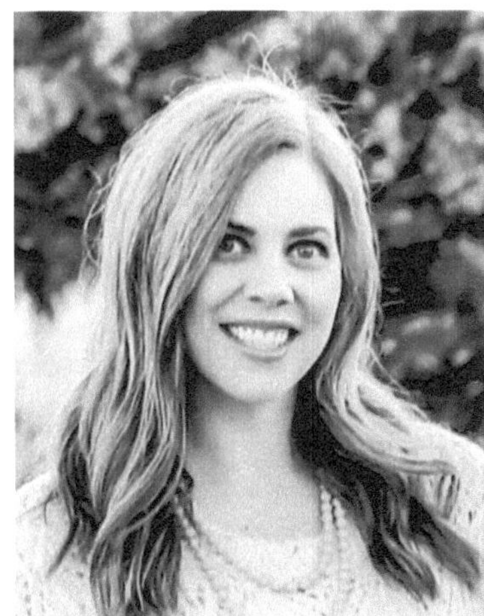

# Getting Started in the Industry

Embarking on a career in the hair styling industry is a journey filled with excitement, creativity, and endless possibilities. As a seasoned stylist, reflecting on my own beginnings in this field brings back memories of passion, determination, and a deep-seated desire to make a difference in people's lives through the art of hair styling.

### Personal Motivation for Becoming a Stylist

My journey into the world of hair styling was ignited by a passion for creativity and a fascination with the transformative power of hair. From a young age, I found joy in experimenting with different hairstyles and helping friends and family members discover their unique looks. Witnessing the boost in their confidence and self-esteem fueled my desire to pursue a career where I could channel my creativity into making a meaningful impact on others.

Beyond the superficial aspect of hair styling, I was drawn to the intimate connection formed between stylist and client. The ability to listen, understand, and translate their desires into beautiful, personalized hairstyles became a driving force in my decision to pursue this path professionally. The prospect of being able to blend my artistic talents with the opportunity to positively influence people's lives was both exhilarating and deeply fulfilling.

### Necessary Skills and Qualifications

Becoming a successful stylist requires more than just a passion for hair; it demands a diverse skill set and a commitment to continuous learning and improvement. While creativity and artistic flair are certainly essential qualities, they must be complemented by technical proficiency and a solid understanding of hair care principles.
In addition to honing their styling techniques, aspiring stylists must also develop strong interpersonal skills to effectively communicate with clients and understand their needs and preferences. Patience, attention to detail, and the ability to work efficiently under pressure are all qualities that contribute to success in this fast-paced industry.

From a qualifications standpoint, obtaining a high school diploma or equivalent is typically the first step towards pursuing a career in hair styling. However, formal training and education from accredited cosmetology schools or vocational training programs are essential for acquiring the

## Getting Started in the Industry

necessary knowledge and skills to excel in this field. These programs cover a wide range of topics, including haircutting, coloring techniques, hair care products, sanitation practices, and business management.

### Finding the Right Training and Education Programs

Choosing the right training and education program is a crucial step in laying the foundation for a successful career in hair styling. With countless options available, it's essential to research and carefully evaluate each program to ensure it aligns with your goals, learning style, and budget.

When considering potential cosmetology schools or training programs, factors such as accreditation, curriculum, faculty expertise, facilities, and job placement assistance should all be taken into account. Visiting campuses, speaking with current students and alumni, and attending informational sessions or open houses can provide valuable insights into the quality of education and overall experience offered by each program.

Ultimately, the goal is to select a program that not only provides comprehensive training in hair styling techniques but also fosters a supportive learning environment conducive to personal and professional growth. Investing in a reputable and respected program sets the stage for a rewarding career and opens doors to endless opportunities within the industry.

### Building a Portfolio and Gaining Experience

Building a portfolio and gaining hands-on experience are essential steps in establishing credibility and showcasing your skills as a stylist. Aspiring stylists can begin by volunteering their services for friends, family members, and local community events to practice their craft and build confidence.

Additionally, seeking out internship or apprenticeship opportunities at reputable salons or studios provides invaluable real-world experience and mentorship from seasoned professionals. This hands-on experience not only allows aspiring stylists to refine their skills but also exposes them to the day-to-day operations of a salon and the intricacies of client interactions.

As their skills progress, aspiring stylists should actively document their work by photographing their creations to compile a comprehensive portfolio. This portfolio serves as a visual representation of their talent, creativity, and versatility and plays a crucial role in attracting potential clients and employers.

In summary, getting started in the hair styling industry requires a combination of passion, dedication, and strategic planning. By identifying their personal motivations, acquiring the necessary skills and qualifications, selecting the right training program, and actively building their portfolio and gaining hands-on experience,

CHAPTER ONE

## Getting Started in the Industry

aspiring stylists can embark on a fulfilling journey towards achieving their career goals in this dynamic and rewarding field.

CHAPTER TWO

# Navigating the Industry Landscape

Navigating the ever-evolving landscape of the hair styling industry requires a keen understanding of industry trends, consumer preferences, and market dynamics. As a seasoned stylist, I've learned that staying ahead of the curve and continuously evolving with the industry are key to remaining competitive and thriving in this dynamic field.

### Understanding Different Hair Styling Techniques and Trends

The world of hair styling is vast and diverse, encompassing a wide range of techniques, trends, and styles. From classic cuts and colors to avant-garde creations, stylists must stay abreast of the latest trends and techniques to meet the diverse needs and preferences of their clients.

Attending industry trade shows, workshops, and seminars is invaluable for staying informed about emerging trends, new products, and cutting-edge techniques. Additionally, following influential stylists and brands on social media platforms and networking with peers allows stylists to stay inspired and connected to the pulse of the industry.

### Identifying Your Niche and Target Market

Identifying a niche and target market is essential for positioning oneself effectively within the industry and attracting the right clientele. Whether it's specializing in bridal hair, men's grooming, or curly hair styling, carving out a distinct niche allows stylists to differentiate themselves from the competition and become sought-after experts in their field.

To identify their niche and target market, stylists should consider factors such as their personal interests and strengths, local market demand, and competition analysis. Conducting market research, surveying potential clients, and analyzing industry trends can provide valuable insights into identifying lucrative niches and target demographics to focus on.

### Researching the Local Market and Competition

Researching the local market and competition is crucial for understanding the competitive landscape and identifying opportunities for growth and differentiation. By conducting thorough market research, stylists can gain insights into local consumer preferences, demographic trends, pricing dynamics, and competitive positioning.

Analyzing competitors' offerings, pricing strategies, marketing tactics, and customer reviews provides valuable benchmarks for identifying gaps in the market and opportunities for differentiation. Leveraging tools such as online directories, social media platforms, and industry publications can also provide valuable insights into local market dynamics and competitor activity.

### Establishing Your Unique Selling Proposition (USP)

Establishing a unique selling proposition (USP) is essential for defining what sets you apart from the competition and communicating your value proposition to potential clients. As a seasoned stylist, I've learned that articulating a compelling USP is key to attracting and retaining loyal clientele in a crowded market.

Your USP should highlight your unique strengths, expertise, and value proposition that differentiate you from other stylists in the area. Whether it's offering personalized consultations, using eco-friendly products, or specializing in a niche service, your USP should resonate with your target market and address their specific needs and preferences.

Crafting a compelling USP requires introspection, market research, and a deep understanding of your target audience. By articulating your unique strengths and value proposition in a clear and compelling manner, you can effectively position yourself as the go-to stylist in your local market and stand out in a competitive industry landscape.

# Setting Up Your Business

Embarking on the journey of setting up your own hair styling business is an exciting yet complex process that requires careful planning, attention to detail, and a clear understanding of the steps involved. As a seasoned stylist who has successfully navigated this process, I understand the importance of laying a strong foundation for your business to thrive.

### Choosing the Right Location for Your Salon or Studio

Choosing the right location for your salon or studio is crucial for the success of your business. The location not only affects your visibility and accessibility to clients but also plays a significant role in shaping your brand image and attracting your target clientele.

When selecting a location, consider factors such as foot traffic, parking availability, proximity to complementary businesses (such as retail shops or restaurants), and the demographic makeup of the surrounding area. Conducting thorough market research and evaluating potential locations against your target market's preferences and needs can help you identify the ideal location for your salon or studio.

### Deciding on a Business Structure (Sole Proprietorship, Partnership, LLC, etc.)

Deciding on the right business structure is an important step in setting up your hair styling business and has implications for your legal and financial responsibilities, tax obligations, and personal liability.

Common business structures for hair styling businesses include sole proprietorships, partnerships, limited liability companies (LLCs), and corporations. Each structure has its own advantages and disadvantages in terms of simplicity, flexibility, liability protection, and tax treatment.

Consider consulting with a legal or financial advisor to determine the most suitable business structure based on your specific circumstances, goals, and preferences. Taking the time to carefully evaluate your options and choose the right business structure sets the stage for long-term success and growth.

### Obtaining Necessary Licenses and Permits

Obtaining the necessary licenses and permits is essential for operating your hair styling business legally and compliantly. Depending on your location and the specific services you offer, you may need to obtain

## Setting Up Your Business

a variety of licenses and permits from local, state, and federal government agencies.

Common licenses and permits required for hair styling businesses may include cosmetology or barbering licenses, business licenses, health department permits, and zoning permits. It's important to research the licensing requirements in your area and ensure that you obtain all necessary permits before opening your salon or studio.

Working with a knowledgeable legal or regulatory advisor can help you navigate the licensing process and ensure that you meet all regulatory requirements. By obtaining the necessary licenses and permits, you can operate your hair styling business with confidence and peace of mind.

**Setting Up Your Salon/Studio Space and Equipment**

Setting up your salon or studio space is an exciting opportunity to bring your vision to life and create a welcoming and professional environment for your clients. From designing the layout and decor to selecting the right equipment and furnishings, every detail contributes to the overall ambiance and client experience.

Consider factors such as the size and layout of your space, the flow of traffic, and the functionality of your equipment when designing your salon or studio. Investing in high-quality equipment and furnishings that align with your brand and service offerings is essential for creating a positive impression and ensuring client comfort and satisfaction.

Additionally, prioritize the implementation of efficient and hygienic practices in your salon or studio to maintain a clean and safe environment for both clients and staff. Establishing protocols for sanitation, disinfection, and sterilization of equipment and surfaces is crucial for upholding professional standards and complying with health and safety regulations.

By carefully planning and executing the setup of your salon or studio space and equipment, you can create an inviting and functional environment that enhances the overall client experience and sets the stage for the success of your hair styling business.

CHAPTER FOUR

# Building Your Brand

Building a strong and recognizable brand is essential for standing out in the competitive hair styling industry and attracting your target clientele. As a seasoned stylist, I've learned that creating a compelling brand identity, establishing a strong online presence, implementing effective marketing strategies, and cultivating relationships with clients are all key components of building a successful brand.

## Creating a Memorable Brand Identity (Name, Logo, Branding Materials)

Crafting a memorable brand identity is the foundation of building a strong brand that resonates with your target audience. Your brand identity encompasses elements such as your salon or studio name, logo, color scheme, typography, and branding materials, all of which should reflect your unique style, personality, and values.

When developing your brand identity, consider factors such as your target market, competitive positioning, and the overall image you want to convey. Collaborating with a professional graphic designer or branding agency can help you create a cohesive and visually appealing brand identity that sets you apart from the competition and leaves a lasting impression on your clients.

## Developing a Strong Online Presence (Website, Social Media Profiles)

In today's digital age, having a strong online presence is essential for reaching and engaging with your target audience. Your website and social media profiles serve as digital storefronts where potential clients can learn more about your services, view your portfolio, and connect with you.

Your website should be professionally designed, easy to navigate, and optimized for mobile devices to provide a seamless user experience. Including high-quality images of your work, client testimonials, and detailed service descriptions can help showcase your expertise and build credibility with potential clients.

In addition to your website, maintaining active and engaging social media profiles on platforms such as Instagram, Facebook, and Pinterest is crucial for reaching a wider audience and building brand awareness. Consistently posting high-quality content, engaging with your followers, and leveraging hashtags and geotags can help boost your visibility and attract new clients.

## Building Your Brand

### Implementing Effective Marketing Strategies (Word of Mouth, Social Media, Advertising)

Implementing effective marketing strategies is essential for promoting your hair styling business and attracting new clients. Word of mouth remains one of the most powerful marketing tools in the industry, so providing exceptional service and cultivating positive relationships with your clients can generate valuable referrals and recommendations.

In addition to word of mouth, leveraging social media platforms and digital advertising can help amplify your marketing efforts and reach a broader audience. Creating targeted social media ads, collaborating with influencers or local businesses, and participating in community events are all effective ways to increase brand visibility and attract new clients.

It's important to track the performance of your marketing strategies and adjust your approach based on what resonates most with your target audience. By experimenting with different tactics and channels, you can identify the most effective ways to promote your hair styling business and achieve your marketing goals.

### Cultivating Relationships with Clients and Building a Loyal Customer Base

Cultivating strong relationships with your clients is essential for building a loyal customer base and fostering repeat business. As a stylist, investing time and effort into building meaningful connections with your clients can lead to long-term relationships and positive word of mouth referrals.

Listening to your clients' needs and preferences, providing personalized recommendations, and delivering exceptional service are all key elements of building trust and loyalty. Additionally, maintaining open and transparent communication, soliciting feedback, and going above and beyond to exceed client expectations can help strengthen your relationships and enhance client satisfaction.

Building a loyal customer base requires ongoing effort and commitment, but the rewards are well worth it. Loyal clients not only provide repeat business and referrals but also serve as brand ambassadors who help promote your business through positive word of mouth and online reviews.

By focusing on building a strong brand identity, establishing a robust online presence, implementing effective marketing strategies, and cultivating meaningful relationships with your clients, you can create a compelling brand that resonates with your target audience and sets the stage for long-term success in the hair styling industry.

CHAPTER FIVE

# Managing Finances

Effective financial management is essential for the success and sustainability of your hair styling business. From setting up a budget and pricing your services competitively to managing cash flow and expenses and tracking income and expenses for tax purposes, mastering the financial aspects of your business is crucial for achieving long-term profitability and growth.

### Setting Up a Budget for Your Business

Setting up a budget is the first step in managing your business finances effectively. A budget serves as a roadmap for allocating your financial resources and helps you plan and prioritize your spending to achieve your business goals.

When creating your budget, consider both fixed expenses (such as rent, utilities, insurance, and equipment costs) and variable expenses (such as supplies, marketing, and staffing). Be realistic and conservative in estimating your revenue and expenses, and regularly review and adjust your budget as needed to reflect changes in your business operations and financial performance.

### Pricing Your Services Competitively

Pricing your services competitively is crucial for attracting clients and generating revenue while ensuring that your business remains profitable. When determining your pricing strategy, consider factors such as your target market, the quality of your services, your level of expertise, and the local market rates.

Researching your competitors' pricing and evaluating the value proposition of your services can help you set prices that are competitive yet reflective of the quality and uniqueness of your offerings. Additionally, consider offering different pricing tiers or packages to cater to different client budgets and preferences while maximizing your revenue potential.

### Managing Cash Flow and Expenses

Managing cash flow is essential for ensuring that your business has enough liquidity to cover its day-to-day operations and financial obligations. To effectively manage cash flow, it's important to monitor your income and expenses closely, anticipate fluctuations in revenue and expenses, and implement strategies to mitigate cash flow gaps.

Maintaining a cash reserve for unexpected expenses and prioritizing timely invoicing and collections can help improve cash flow and liquidity. Additionally,

## Managing Finances

negotiating favorable payment terms with suppliers and vendors and implementing efficient inventory management practices can help optimize cash flow and reduce expenses.

### Tracking Income and Expenses for Tax Purposes

Accurate record-keeping and tracking of income and expenses are essential for fulfilling your tax obligations and maximizing tax deductions for your hair styling business. Keeping detailed records of all income sources, expenses, and business transactions throughout the year can streamline tax preparation and help you take advantage of potential tax deductions and credits.

Utilizing accounting software or hiring a professional bookkeeper can help simplify the process of tracking income and expenses and ensure compliance with tax regulations. Additionally, staying informed about tax laws and regulations relevant to your business and seeking guidance from a tax professional can help you optimize your tax strategy and minimize your tax liability.

By proactively managing your business finances, including setting up a budget, pricing your services competitively, managing cash flow and expenses, and tracking income and expenses for tax purposes, you can establish a solid financial foundation for your hair styling business and achieve long-term success and profitability.

CHAPTER SIX

# Providing Exceptional Service

As a seasoned stylist, providing exceptional service is not just a goal but a fundamental aspect of building a successful hair styling business. Understanding and exceeding client needs and expectations, developing excellent communication and interpersonal skills, providing personalized consultations and recommendations, and delivering high-quality services while maintaining professional standards are all key components of delivering exceptional service.

**Understanding Client Needs and Expectations**

Understanding your clients' needs and expectations is essential for delivering personalized and satisfying hair styling experiences. Take the time to listen actively and attentively to your clients' preferences, concerns, and desired outcomes during consultations. Ask probing questions to gain a deeper understanding of their lifestyle, hair care routine, and styling preferences.

By empathizing with your clients' needs and expectations, you can tailor your services to meet their specific requirements and exceed their expectations. Whether it's recommending suitable hairstyles, discussing color options, or addressing concerns about hair health and maintenance, demonstrating genuine care and attention to detail fosters trust and loyalty with your clients.

**Developing Excellent Communication and Interpersonal Skills**

Developing excellent communication and interpersonal skills is essential for building rapport with your clients and creating a positive and comfortable salon experience. Effective communication involves more than just verbal exchanges; it also encompasses nonverbal cues, active listening, and empathy.

Maintain open and transparent communication with your clients throughout the styling process, explaining each step and discussing any concerns or preferences they may have. Practice active listening by paying attention to your clients' verbal and nonverbal cues and responding empathetically to their needs and feedback.

Additionally, hone your interpersonal skills by cultivating a warm and welcoming demeanor, demonstrating professionalism and respect, and fostering a supportive and inclusive salon environment. Building strong relationships with your clients based on trust, mutual respect, and effective communication lays the foundation for long-term client satisfaction and loyalty.

### Providing Personalized Consultations and Recommendations

Providing personalized consultations and recommendations is essential for delivering tailored and satisfying hair styling experiences that meet your clients' unique needs and preferences. Start each client interaction with a thorough consultation to assess their hair type, texture, face shape, lifestyle, and styling goals.

During the consultation, take the time to educate your clients about suitable hairstyles, color options, and styling techniques that complement their features and align with their personal style. Provide honest and constructive feedback based on your expertise and experience while considering your clients' preferences and concerns.

Offer personalized recommendations for at-home hair care products, styling techniques, and maintenance routines to help your clients maintain their desired look between salon visits. By empowering your clients with knowledge and guidance, you demonstrate your commitment to their satisfaction and success beyond the salon chair.

### Delivering High-Quality Services and Maintaining Professional Standards

Delivering high-quality services and maintaining professional standards are non-negotiable aspects of providing exceptional service as a stylist. Uphold industry best practices and hygiene standards to ensure the safety and well-being of your clients and staff.

Invest in continuous education and training to stay updated on the latest trends, techniques, and products in the hair styling industry. Strive for excellence in every aspect of your work, from precision cutting and coloring to styling and finishing techniques.

Additionally, prioritize the use of high-quality products and tools that align with your clients' needs and preferences and contribute to superior results. By delivering consistently excellent services and upholding professional standards, you demonstrate your dedication to providing exceptional experiences that exceed your clients' expectations and foster long-term loyalty.

In summary, providing exceptional service as a stylist requires a combination of understanding client needs and expectations, developing excellent communication and interpersonal skills, providing personalized consultations and recommendations, and delivering high-quality services while maintaining professional standards. By prioritizing these key components, you can create memorable and satisfying hair styling experiences that leave a lasting impression on your clients and set your business apart in the competitive salon industry.

CHAPTER SEVEN

# Growing Your Business

Growing your hair styling business requires strategic planning, innovation, and a customer-centric approach. As a seasoned stylist, I've learned that expanding your service offerings, hiring and training staff, expanding your client base through referrals and networking, and leveraging technology to streamline operations are all essential components of achieving sustainable growth and success.

**Expanding Your Service Offerings (e.g., Additional Treatments, Products)**

Expanding your service offerings is a strategic way to attract new clients, increase revenue, and differentiate your hair styling business from competitors. Consider introducing additional treatments and services that complement your core offerings, such as hair treatments, extensions, or special occasion styling.

Research market trends and client preferences to identify new services and products that align with your target market's needs and preferences. Collaborating with reputable brands and suppliers to offer high-quality products and treatments can enhance the value proposition of your salon and attract clients seeking premium services.

Promote your new offerings through targeted marketing campaigns, social media, and word of mouth referrals to generate excitement and drive demand. By continuously innovating and expanding your service offerings, you can position your hair styling business as a one-stop destination for all of your clients' beauty needs.

**Hiring and Training Staff (If Applicable)**

As your hair styling business grows, hiring and training staff can help you expand your capacity, improve service quality, and scale your operations. When hiring staff, prioritize candidates who share your passion for hair styling, possess excellent technical skills, and demonstrate strong interpersonal abilities.

Invest in comprehensive training programs to onboard new staff members and ensure they adhere to your salon's standards and protocols. Provide ongoing education and professional development opportunities to help your team stay updated on the latest trends, techniques, and products in the industry.

Empower your staff to deliver exceptional customer service by fostering a positive and supportive work environment that encourages collaboration, creativity, and continuous improvement. By building a talented and cohesive team, you can enhance the overall client experience and position your salon for long-term success.

### Expanding Your Client Base Through Referrals and Networking

Expanding your client base through referrals and networking is a cost-effective and powerful way to grow your hair styling business. Encourage satisfied clients to refer their friends, family members, and colleagues to your salon by offering incentives such as referral discounts or loyalty rewards.

Participate in local community events, industry trade shows, and networking groups to connect with potential clients and build relationships with other professionals in the beauty and wellness industry. Collaborating with complementary businesses, such as spas, makeup artists, or bridal shops, can also help you expand your client base through cross-promotion and referrals.

Leverage social media platforms, online reviews, and testimonials to showcase your work, engage with your audience, and build credibility and trust with potential clients. By actively engaging in networking and referral programs, you can attract new clients and foster long-term relationships that drive repeat business and referrals.

### Leveraging Technology to Streamline Operations and Enhance Customer Experience

Leveraging technology is essential for streamlining operations, improving efficiency, and enhancing the customer experience in your hair styling business. Invest in salon management software or booking systems to streamline appointment scheduling, manage client records, and track inventory.

Utilize social media platforms, email marketing, and online booking tools to communicate with clients, promote your services, and offer convenient booking options. Implement digital tools and applications to streamline payment processing, automate appointment reminders, and gather client feedback.

Integrate technology into the salon experience by offering amenities such as Wi-Fi access, digital magazines, or entertainment options to enhance client comfort and satisfaction. Embrace innovative tools and devices, such as hair analysis systems or virtual makeover apps, to personalize consultations and recommend tailored treatments.

By leveraging technology to streamline operations and enhance the customer experience, you can improve salon efficiency, increase client satisfaction, and position your hair styling business for continued growth and success in a competitive market.

# Expanding Your Service Offerings

Expanding your service offerings is a strategic approach to diversifying your revenue streams and meeting the evolving needs and preferences of your clientele. By introducing additional treatments and products, you can attract new clients, retain existing ones, and maximize the lifetime value of each customer.

Consider conducting market research and client surveys to identify gaps in your current service offerings and areas of unmet demand. Look for opportunities to expand into complementary services that align with your salon's brand and expertise. For example, if you specialize in hair styling, you could consider adding services such as hair treatments, scalp massages, or hair extensions to enhance your clients' experience.

Collaborating with reputable brands and suppliers can also help you enhance your service offerings with high-quality products and treatments. Partnering with skincare or beauty brands to offer facials, waxing, or makeup services can attract clients seeking a holistic beauty experience.

When introducing new services, invest in training and certification for yourself and your staff to ensure competency and quality delivery. Promote your expanded service menu through various marketing channels, such as your website, social media platforms, email newsletters, and in-salon signage, to generate interest and drive bookings.

**Hiring and Training Staff (If Applicable)**

As your hair styling business grows, hiring and training staff can help you scale your operations and meet the increasing demand for your services. When hiring new staff members, consider their technical skills, experience, and cultural fit with your salon's values and brand identity.

Create a structured onboarding process to familiarize new hires with your salon's policies, procedures, and service standards. Provide comprehensive training on haircutting techniques, coloring methods, customer service protocols, and product knowledge to ensure consistency and quality across your team.

Encourage ongoing professional development and skill enhancement through workshops, seminars, and advanced training programs. Investing in your staff's growth and development not only improves service quality but also fosters employee engagement and loyalty.

also fosters employee engagement and loyalty.

Promote a positive work culture and team collaboration by recognizing and rewarding employee contributions, fostering open communication, and providing opportunities for career advancement. By building a talented and motivated team, you can enhance the overall client experience and position your salon for long-term success.

### Expanding Your Client Base Through Referrals and Networking

Expanding your client base through referrals and networking is a powerful and cost-effective way to grow your hair styling business. Encourage satisfied clients to refer their friends, family members, and colleagues to your salon by offering incentives such as referral discounts, loyalty rewards, or complimentary services.

Actively engage in networking opportunities within your local community and industry to build relationships with potential clients and referral partners. Attend networking events, join professional associations, and participate in community activities to expand your network and increase your visibility.

Collaborate with complementary businesses, such as wedding planners, event venues, or photographers, to tap into new client demographics and referral channels. Offer joint promotions or cross-promotional opportunities to incentivize referrals and strengthen partnerships.

Leverage the power of social media and online reviews to showcase your work, engage with your audience, and build credibility with potential clients. Encourage satisfied clients to leave positive reviews and testimonials on platforms such as Google My Business, Yelp, and Facebook to enhance your salon's online reputation and attract new clients.

### Leveraging Technology to Streamline Operations and Enhance Customer Experience

Incorporating technology into your salon operations can streamline processes, improve efficiency, and enhance the overall customer experience. Invest in salon management software or booking systems to automate appointment scheduling, manage client records, and track inventory in real-time.

Offer online booking options through your salon's website or mobile app to provide convenience and flexibility for clients to book appointments anytime, anywhere. Implement automated appointment reminders via email or text messaging to reduce no-shows and keep clients informed about their upcoming appointments.

Utilize social media platforms, email marketing, and digital advertising to promote your salon services, share client testimonials, and engage with your audience. Create engaging content, such as tutorials, behind-

## Expanding Your Services

the-scenes videos, or before-and-after transformations, to showcase your expertise and personality and attract potential clients.

Integrate digital payment options, such as mobile payment apps or contactless payments, to provide a seamless and secure checkout experience for clients. Explore innovative technologies, such as virtual consultations, augmented reality hair color simulations, or virtual reality salon tours, to enhance the client experience and differentiate your salon from competitors.

By leveraging technology to streamline operations and enhance the customer experience, you can improve salon efficiency, increase client satisfaction, and drive business growth in today's digital age.

# Overcoming Challenges

As a seasoned stylist, I've encountered and overcome various challenges throughout my career. Whether it's dealing with competition and market saturation, handling difficult clients or situations, managing stress and burnout, or adapting to industry changes and trends, overcoming these challenges requires resilience, adaptability, and a proactive approach to problem-solving.

**Dealing with Competition and Market Saturation**

In the competitive landscape of the hair styling industry, dealing with competition and market saturation is a common challenge. To overcome this challenge, focus on differentiating your salon by emphasizing your unique selling points, such as exceptional customer service, specialized expertise, or innovative service offerings.

Conduct a competitive analysis to identify gaps in the market and opportunities for differentiation. Consider niche markets or underserved demographics that you can target with specialized services or promotional campaigns.

Build strong relationships with your existing clients by providing exceptional service and cultivating loyalty through loyalty programs, referral incentives, and personalized experiences. Encourage satisfied clients to leave positive reviews and testimonials to enhance your salon's reputation and attract new clients.

**Handling Difficult Clients or Situations**

Handling difficult clients or situations is an inevitable part of running a hair styling business. When faced with challenging clients or situations, remain calm, professional, and empathetic. Listen actively to the client's concerns and address them with patience and understanding.

Communicate clearly and transparently with the client to manage their expectations and find a mutually satisfactory solution. Offer alternatives or compromises when appropriate, and strive to turn a negative experience into a positive one by going above and beyond to exceed the client's expectations.

Establish clear policies and boundaries to manage difficult clients and maintain a respectful and professional salon environment. Train your staff on conflict resolution techniques and empower them to handle challenging situations effectively and diplomatically.

CHAPTER NINE

# Overcoming Challenges

### Managing Stress and Burnout

Managing stress and burnout is essential for maintaining your well-being and performance as a stylist. To prevent burnout, prioritize self-care and establish healthy work-life balance practices. Take regular breaks, exercise regularly, and engage in activities that promote relaxation and rejuvenation.

Delegate tasks and responsibilities to your team members or consider outsourcing non-essential tasks to lighten your workload. Set realistic goals and expectations for yourself and your salon, and avoid overcommitting to projects or appointments that could lead to burnout.

Practice stress management techniques such as mindfulness meditation, deep breathing exercises, or yoga to reduce stress and promote mental clarity and focus. Seek support from friends, family members, or professional mentors to discuss challenges and brainstorm solutions.

### Adapting to Industry Changes and Trends

Adapting to industry changes and trends is essential for staying relevant and competitive in the fast-paced hair styling industry. Keep abreast of emerging trends, techniques, and technologies by attending industry trade shows, workshops, and continuing education programs.

Invest in ongoing professional development and training for yourself and your team to stay updated on the latest industry developments and enhance your skills and expertise. Experiment with new services, products, and marketing strategies to stay ahead of the curve and attract new clients.

Embrace innovation and creativity in your salon operations and service offerings to differentiate yourself from competitors and appeal to modern consumers. Leverage social media platforms and digital marketing tools to showcase your work, engage with your audience, and stay connected with current and potential clients.

By proactively addressing and overcoming challenges such as competition and market saturation, difficult clients or situations, stress and burnout, and industry changes and trends, you can position yourself and your salon for long-term success and growth in the dynamic and competitive hair styling industry.

CHAPTER TEN

# Conclusion

As I reflect on my journey as a stylist and business owner, I'm filled with a sense of gratitude for the opportunities, challenges, and growth that have shaped my career in the hair styling industry. From humble beginnings to establishing my own salon and building a loyal clientele, my journey has been a testament to the passion, dedication, and resilience required to succeed in this dynamic field.

**Reflection on Your Journey as a Stylist and Business Owner**

Throughout my career, I've experienced the highs and lows of being a stylist and business owner. From mastering new techniques and trends to navigating industry challenges and overcoming setbacks, each experience has contributed to my growth and evolution as a professional.

I've learned the importance of continuously honing my craft, staying updated on industry developments, and adapting to changing consumer preferences and market dynamics. Building strong relationships with clients, fostering a positive salon culture, and prioritizing professionalism and quality have been the cornerstones of my success as a stylist and business owner.

**Encouragement and Advice for Aspiring Stylists**

To aspiring stylists embarking on their own journey in the hair styling industry, I offer the following encouragement and advice:

**Follow Your Passion:** Pursue a career in hair styling because it's your passion and calling. Embrace your creativity, curiosity, and love for beauty and aesthetics as you embark on this fulfilling journey.

**Invest in Education and Training:** Commit to lifelong learning and professional development. Seek out reputable training programs, workshops, and mentorships to enhance your skills, expand your knowledge, and stay updated on industry trends.

**Build Your Portfolio:** Invest time and effort into building a strong portfolio that showcases your skills, creativity, and unique style. High-quality photos and client testimonials are invaluable tools for attracting new clients and establishing your credibility as a stylist.

**Network and Collaborate:** Build relationships with fellow stylists, industry professionals, and potential mentors. Networking opportunities and collaborative partnerships can open doors to new opportunities, referrals, and growth.

**Embrace Resilience and Adaptability:** The hair styling industry is dynamic and ever-changing. Embrace challenges as opportunities for growth, stay adaptable to changing

## Overcoming Challenges

trends and technologies, and remain resilient in the face of setbacks.

### Final Thoughts and Closing Remarks

In closing, I want to express my gratitude to all the clients, mentors, and colleagues who have supported me on my journey as a stylist and business owner. Their trust, encouragement, and feedback have been invaluable sources of inspiration and motivation.

To my fellow stylists and aspiring professionals in the hair styling industry, remember that success is not defined by accolades or achievements, but by the lives we touch, the relationships we build, and the passion we bring to our craft every day.

May your journey in the hair styling industry be filled with creativity, fulfillment, and endless opportunities for growth and success. As you embark on this exciting adventure, remember to stay true to yourself, embrace challenges with grace and resilience, and always strive for excellence in everything you do.

Thank you, and here's to a bright and beautiful future in the world of hair styling.

www.ingramcontent.com/pod-product-compliance
Lightning Source LLC
Chambersburg PA
CBHW051409250726
48656CB00006B/2355

* 9 7 9 8 3 2 7 2 4 2 9 7 5 *